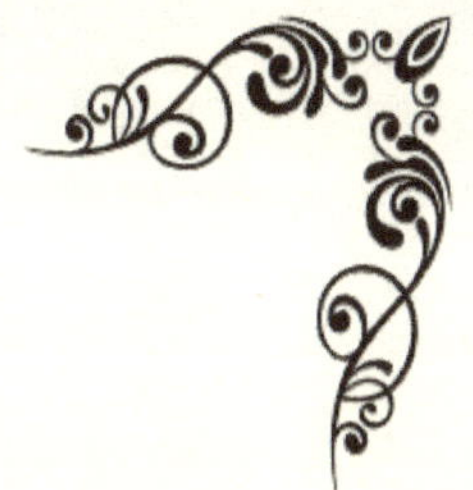

Foreword

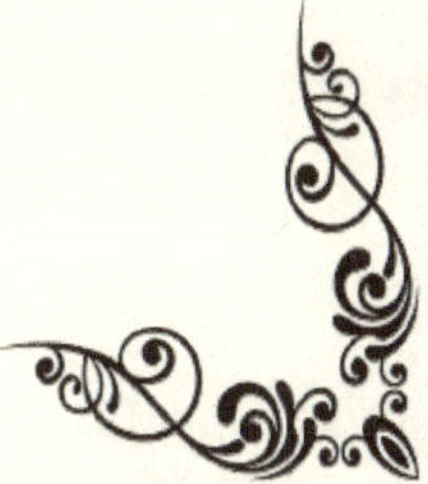

Foreword

Lucid dreaming is the ability to observe and/or control dreams. It is an altered state of consciousness when you realize you are dreaming and you have the ability to switch your brain into being awake, while inside a dream.

Your dreams become exceptionally vivid and also feel unusually real. It is a safe and natural state, and it is a skill that can be cultivated by ANYONE as long as they are willing to demonstrate practice and persistence.

If you know anything about lucid dreaming, you'll know that there is ALWAYS more to do.

You can always have a more vivid dream, or slightly LONGER in the dream, and there's always things

you WISH you did, once you've woken up.

That's where supplements come in. Through supplementation, we're able to alter our brain chemistry, and have a huge effect on dreaming and the dreaming mind.

This means we're able to massively improve the lucid dreaming experience, when we know how to do it through supplements, herbs and substances.

Most people have accidentally become lucid at some point, but it is also possible (and very common) to experience this phenomenon intentionally. Some say it should really be called "conscious dreaming" because it's the change in consciousness that defines the experience. Whatever the case, practitioners agree that it is an altogether life changing

experience once you learn how to do it
with some ease.

How does it work?

Why would anyone want to do this?

*Plenty of reasons! The rewards are
endless.*

Would you like to have dreams that allow
yourself to explore your subconscious
mind? How about have the ability to
control the outcome of your dream?

With lucid dreaming, your senses come
alive and you're able to begin a journey of
a deeper understanding of yourself on
every level.

It's worth taking some to understand
what lucid dreaming is NOT, but we will
spend more time discussing what it
actually is and how to experience it.

In a lucid dream you're in REM (rapid eye movement) sleep, but part of your brain has become reactivated while you're dreaming allowing you to experience a dream consciously.

It's not JUST a very vivid dream, even though lucid dreams ARE often vivid experiences. It's also not an out-of-body experience or an astral projection.

Lucid dreams are dominated by the personal mind state of the dreamer, but out-of-body experiences and astral projection take us to whole new realms and areas of discussion.

When dreamers are aware of their dreams, they can affect their own overall well-being. As a lucid dreamer gains experience and learns more, he or she can use lucid dreaming as a way of developing wisdom, exploring other realms and improving their overall quality of life.

Many also report improved creativity and confidence.

Research on lucid dreaming suggests that it can be used as a treatment for recurring nightmares. It can also have **emotional benefits** like gaining closure from difficult and/or traumatic memories.

I find this sort of thing amazing and interesting to research. I'm sure you'll agree that we're still just at the start of this topic, and I don't think we'll ever know EVERYTHING about lucid dreaming or our own brains.

In addition, lucid dreaming can help you experience altered states of consciousness. Experienced lucid dreamers say that connecting the conscious with the unconscious opens up whole new worlds and life becomes deeper and more meaningful.

How can supplements help you lucid dream?

Supplements are a powerful tool for enhancing lucid dreaming (and our lives in general) and they are used to supplement missing elements in your diet.

This term is broad based; however, the Food and Drug Administration (FDA) defines a supplement as "a product taken by mouth that contains a 'dietary ingredient' intended to supplement the diet.

By the way, we've also collected a huge list of all of these lucid dreaming supplements and made it easy to buy them, along with giving you some discounts on them!

At the very end of this book is a secret link and details on how to get

discounts on all of these supplements.

The 'dietary ingredients' in these products may include: vitamins, minerals, herbs or other botanicals, amino acids, and substances such as enzymes, organ tissues, glandulars, and metabolites." .
Now for some boring stuff..

It's important to remember that not all supplements are regulated by a governing agency to attest to their safety.

Always consult a medical professional, dietician or holistic practitioner before using new supplements.

Supplement labels can sometimes be deceiving. However, if you do your homework, using supplements can be extremely beneficial for lucid dreaming.

General tips for using supplements before we go any further:

- Always research the product yourself. Search online and see what reputable professionals are saying about the supplement and make sure their claims are supported by scientific research.

- Research supplement manufacturers and only buy from reputable sources. There are many scam artists and companies selling supplements on the market. Without regulation, it is easy for manufacturers to make false claims about what is in a supplement bottle, and what it can do.

- Do not exceed the recommended dose when taking supplements. This may cause serious harm.

Supplements may include also include energy bars and drinks or sports nutrition products.

Supplements should be used in addition to a healthy and well-balanced diet and should not replace good eating choices. If you have questions, again, it's always wise to seek professional counsel about how to use supplements safely.

It's also important to note that the information in this book is NOT approved or reviewed by a medical professional and is ONLY the summary and interpretation of my own research and understanding of these supplements and how they work.

For the most part I've tried to summarise existing research that's already been done, or I'm consolidating information that's already out there about these supplements. I'm not a trained medical

How do lucid dreaming supplements REALLY work?

Understanding the neurochemistry behind lucid dreaming is important if you want to have an optimal experience. Lucid dreaming begins in the brain; therefore, it's important to understand how the brain affects the dreaming process.

If you want to take your dreams to a new realm, it's important to learn how to maximize results by balancing your neurotransmitters.

A neurotransmitter is essentially a chemical substance released by the ends of your nerve fibres. It's a 'spark' that transfers information and substances through your body and nerves.

The two main neurotransmitters involved in lucid dreaming are Norepinephrine and Acytelcholine.

Norepinephrine is what helps you to gain control of the dream, and Acytelcholine is what aids in accessing your memories.

Memories are important for consciousness and we become unconscious during our dreams because we lose access to our memories.

Norepinephrine accelerates the Rapid Eye Movement (REM) sleep phase and increases alertness.

Several options are available on the market but it's important to remember that these should be taken after four hours of sleep. In other words, you will have to set an alarm in order to wake up in the middle of your sleep cycle.

Acetylcholine helps connect your thoughts to your memories and helps with REM sleep. There are two ways to increase acetylcholine. Acetylcholene can be promoted by either increasing the production of acetylcholine or by slowing the loss of acetylcholine.

Interestingly Acetylcholene levels are at their highest during the last stages of sleep when your REM sleep is longest as well. So it seems very obvious that the BEST time to lucid dream is actually in that window, between 4-7Am in the morning.

That window will change depending on when you usually wake up, but in general you'll want to target the part of the night that's about 2-3 hours BEFORE you normally wake up naturally. For most people this is about 5-8AM.

The link between this neurotransmitter Acetylcholene and memory is also strong.

It was found that in people with Alzihemers, their Acetylcholene producing cells were among the first to die, suggesting that it's strongly linked to memory and mental clarity.

It's been said numerous times that just increasing the levels of Acetylcholene in your body will give you more vivid dreams, but don't start doing it yet! If you just storm in trying to increase Acetylcholene levels, you'll also get nightmares and more vivid bad dreams.

You've got to use a balanced approach as we'll cover in a minute, and many lucid supplements HAVE that balanced approach involving boosting Acetylcholene levels safely.

There are also lots of foods that can naturally boost Acetylcholene levels and give you more vivid dreams but this guide is focused on supplements as opposed to diet for the most part.

As a rule of thumb, you can get a lot of benefits from eating a vegan or mainly plant based diet, and that includes boosting your Acetylcholene levels to your memory improves.

There are of course LOTS of substances and supplements that you could use in lucid dreaming, and we're going to cover individual supplements later on.

There are things like Huperzine A for example which is also a prominent lucid pill but we'll cover that later. First, let's look at how your sleep cycles work:

How your sleep cycle works (99% get this wrong)

An average night of sleep is divided into several REM (rapid eye movement) and four stages of non-REM cycles.

Now you probably already know that dreams and lucid dreams happen during your REM sleep, specifically the LATER stages of REM sleep in the early hours of the morning. In each stage of sleep, your brain is operating at a different brain wave frequency.

Stage one of non-REM is the stage of beginning to drift off where one is between sleeping and waking.

In stage two the brain continues to slow down with only occasional bursts of activity. Then everything begins to shut down in stages three and four, and the brain moves into a slow brain wave state, and heart and breathing rates drop significantly.

It usually takes about 70 minutes of non-REM sleep to experience the first period of REM, and it lasts a mere five minutes. To clarify, REM sleep only lasts 5 minutes at the very START of your nights sleep.

A complete sleep cycle is 90 minutes and it repeats about five times throughout a night. However, non-REM stages shorten, and the REM periods grow leading to a 40-minute REM stage just before waking. The difference is massive, 5 minutes at the start of the night leading to up to 40 minutes of REM towards the end of your sleep.

It's important to know this as it means you can start to think about the BEST time to take supplements.

It's not always right before bed as many people think. As I said, the first stage of sleep only actually gives you about 5 minutes of REM sleep, so it's unlikely you'll have a lucid dream then.

It's better to wait until the early hours of the morning when your REM sleep stages are longer, and you're more likely to become lucid as well.

That's why (as we'll cover soon) the best time to take most lucid dreaming pills is actually in the early hours of the morning, for example 4AM.

What is the Rapid Eye Movement (REM) sleep cycle?

The REM sleep cycle is the fifth and final stage of sleep and it is the most eventful (and arguably the most important) stage for dreaming and resting.

This stage of sleep result in dreams and it is also important for a healthy brain and for long-term memory capacity. And most importantly – this is when lucid dreaming happens!

The REM cycle is characterised by distinctive eye movements during sleep. It's also known as "paradoxical sleep" because the brain becomes more active during REM sleep than when a person is awake. how can this be, if the person is dreaming?

Well it's not known, but it's interesting to note that your brain can be MORE active when you're dreaming than when you're awake. That might explain how dreams can be so complex and vivid.

It has been theorized that the brain may be reacting to different types of imagery and that this is why there are rapid eye movements. It could literally be your eyes looking around the dream scene.

In fact several lucid dreaming studies have been performed in which participants 'prove' they're lucid by falling asleep, getting lucid and then looking from side to side in their lucid dreams, in a pre determined pattern.

The people watching them sleep were then able to track their eye movements and prove they were in fact lucid dreaming.

REM also causes most of the muscles (except for the diaphragm and the heart) to be temporarily paralyzed from the chin down (explaining why we're still able to move our eyes during this period of sleep). Researchers suspect that this is so that the body does not act out the content of dreams.

Other physiological occurrences during REM include a rapid an increased heartbeat which may be a physiological response to dream content and lower body temperature that is a result of circadian influences.

During a full night of uninterrupted sleep, the brain has an opportunity to remove neurotoxins which is helpful for the lucid dreaming experience.

The REM rebound effect: 10X more vivid dreams

The REM rebound effect is when a person someone is deprived of sleep for a short period of time, but then when they finally get to sleep, there is increased brain activity, and much longer REM sleep.

As a result, dreams become more intense and vivid and the whole experience seems to last much longer and be more intense.

Unfortunately, the only way to study this, is by putting a subject through intense sleep deprivation or by taking a drug that's a 'REM suppressant' like cannabis or alcohol.

You might have even experienced this yourself randomly, and noticed that if you drink a certain amount and then go to sleep thinking about things, you'll have intense and often lucid dreams. It only works if you drink the right amount that can be digested during your sleep.

If you drink LOTS the night before then you'll suppress ALL of your REM sleep. But drink just the right amount, and then maybe have a snack before bed to soak up the alcohol, and you'll have vivid dreams.

When researchers are studying this phenomenon they follow the electroencephalogram tracing and when subjects begin to move toward REM sleep they are woken up. When people are deprived of REM sleep, there is a lot of pressure for them to return to the REM state, and it gradually builds.

REM rebound shows that specific sleep stages are NEEDED by the brain. In some marine animals, when one brain hemisphere is lacking REM sleep, only the deprived hemisphere will go into REM rebound, and the other hemisphere won't be affected.

This phenomenon is frequently seen in people who take sleeping pills and it is also seen in the first few nights after patients with sleep apnea are placed on a CPAP machine.

Many antidepressants, particularly selective serotonin re-uptake inhibitors (SSRIs), inhibit REM sleep and may also cause REM rebound. All of that being said though, alcohol is probably not the healthiest way to lucid dream, and it certainly isn't sustainable to just get drunk every night, in the hopes of becoming lucid.

The best way of approaching this is just to bear in mind that if you were going to have a drink anyway, there's a good chance you can turn that night into a lucid dream if you just hold the intention in your mind as you go to sleep.

Maybe put a note above your bed on somewhere you'll be able to see it that says 'you'll become lucid tonight' and just stare at it before you go to sleep.

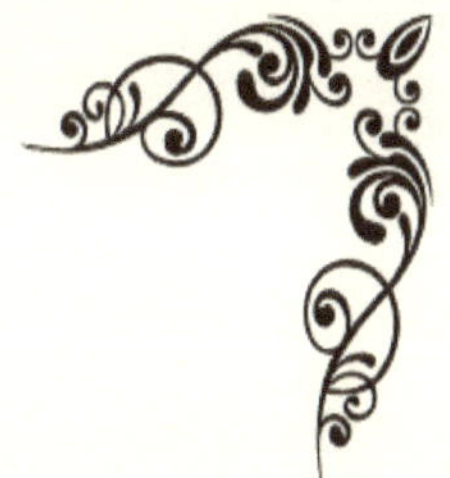

Common THEORIES
for why we dream

Common theories on WHY we dream

Human beings have been theorizing about why we actually dream for centuries. Ancient people believed that we dream in order to receive spiritual wisdom.

Psychoanalyst Sigmund Freud, perhaps the most famous dream theorist of all time, speculated that dreams are the gateway to the unconscious. However, we've come a long way since Freud's time and different dream theories are commonly discussed now.

While many theories have been proposed, no single consensus has emerged. Considering the enormous amount of time we spend in a dreaming state, the fact that researchers do not yet understand the purpose of dreams may seem baffling. However, it is important to consider that science is still unraveling the exact purpose and function of sleep itself.

Freuds theory

Freud believed that dreams are about the unconscious mind and much of his research focused on repressed sexual desire. He theorized that the brain protects us from disturbing memories, through repression.

While Freud was certainly a pioneer in his field, we now know that he had little understanding of REM sleep and the ramifications of this stage of sleep.

Freud said that dreams are a way to process subconscious emotions while asleep. Without dreams, we'd be constantly disturbed by our deepest emotions.

John Allan Hobsons theory

John Allan Hobson studies neurochemicals in the brain and the effect of electrical impulses on the brain. Hobson believes Freud had too ominous of a theory about dreams. Hobson believes in psychological meaning to dreams.

However, he believes that the meaning isn't buried deeply in the subconscious as Freud did. Hobson adopted a Jungian approach. In other words, he believes that dreams can actually be quite transparent.

We may dream to organize our minds. Think of all of the information that we receive during the course of a typical day. Perhaps dreams are nature's way of helping us sort through unneeded information.

While this theory hasn't been proven by research, some believe dreaming helps us declutter our minds and that it aids in maximizing learning.

Critics say that this theory amounts to little more than comparing human beings to a computer storage system and it is not a very prevalent theory.

There is some research to back up the idea that dreams are related to how we form memories. Studies indicate that as we're learning new things in our daily life, dreams increase while we sleep.

Participants in a dream study who were taking a language course showed more dream activity than those who were not actively engaged in the course. The idea that we use our dreams convert short-term memories into long-term memories has gained some traction in recent years.

Fight or Flight

It's interesting to note that the amygdala is the most active part of the brain during dreams.

The amygdala is associated with our 'survival instinct' and the fight-or-flight response. One theory suggests that because the amygdala is more active during sleep, it may be a way of preparing to deal with real danger.

However, the brainstem sends out signals during REM sleep that relax the muscles. As a result, we don't act out the physicality of our dreams.

I think we can't rule out the possibility that through dreaming, our bodies and minds are actually preparing to deal with things in the real world. For example, think about a dangerous situation like a physical confrontation or being chased by a dog.

If we've already had loads of dreams about that situation, we're much more likely to know how to respond and be able to deal with it. Our brains have prepared for it and we're not so worried any more. Or at least, we're far LESS worried than we would be if we'd NEVER had a dream about it.

We'll never know for sure but it's an interesting theory. And don't worry, we're getting onto the supplement guides very soon, it's just useful to have some context and background.

Dreaming In Order To Solve Problems

Some researchers postulate that we dream as a way of working through dilemmas that we are not able to solve in our waking life and that our dreams help us look at issues that go unnoticed during the day.

The term "sleeping on it" may apply here since that is a term often used to having a fresh perspective after a good night's sleep. Critics of this theory suggest that if the purpose of dreams is to solve problems, shouldn't we have better recall of our dreams?

Dreaming As a Way of Coping With Trauma

This theory is more commonly accepted among dream theories. Because of the intensity of emotions surrounding trauma, dreams can be a way of processing deep emotional pain.

Dreaming about a traumatic event can help a person make sense of an event and perhaps even prevent the event from happening again.

Another theory is that dreams are a reflection of our emotions. During the day, our brains are working hard to make connections.

Some have postulated that at night everything slows down and since it's not required to focus on anything during sleep, our brains relax and make looser connections.

It's during sleep that the experiences and emotions of the our waking life play out in our dreams. If something is bothering you during the day, you will likely dream about it.

There's also a theory that dreams don't really serve any purpose at all and that they're just a meaningless byproduct of the brain while we sleep. We know that the rear portion of our brain is very active during REM sleep when most dreaming occurs.

Some suggest that it's just the brain winding down from the day and that dreams are random and meaningless. Unfortunately, as long as the brain remains such a mystery, we probably won't be able to say with absolute certainty what purpose dreams serve.

Lucid SUPPLEMENTS
Guides (Specific)

Lucid Dream Supplements: Complete guide

Galantamine: Inception juice

Galantamine hydrobromide is a compound found in many plant species. Most commonly it is found in daffodils, however, it is also found in the red spider lily (which is why it's one of the main ingredients in Claridream) and the snowdrop plant.

It is often used to enhance memory in Alzheimer and Dementia patients. Patients who suffer from these conditions say that galantamine improves both short and long term memory as well as makes dreams appear more vivid and intense.

It makes sense then that galantamine would have a positive effect for lucid dreaming, A chemical called acetyl cholinesterase breaks down a neurotransmitter called acetylcholine.

Galantamine stops this from occurring which increases acetylcholine. As a result, there is higher memory allowing for improved dream recall as well as more ability to dream lucidly.

People tend to find that galantamine based lucid dreaming supplements can be a bit intense, and hard to digest. For this reason, whenever you're taking a supplement with Galantamine in it, try taking a cube of ginger or other digestive aid, as it will make it less rough. Also start with a really low dose and go up from there.

Having swallowed a pill, galantamine will take full effect within an hour or so. In order to enhance your lucid dreaming, the right dosage is between 4-8

milligrams which is way less than with Alzheimer patients.

REM cycles have been shown to occur more frequently past midnight. It is therefore best to take galantamine at midnight to take advantage of this. Swallowing the pill before this time can result in the sleep paralysis and nightmares as we saw above.

I'd actually take that one step further and say that it's really ONLY worth taking galantamine in the early hours of the morning. You've got to wake yourself up super early and take it.

The problem with that is that because it's already fairly intense to digest and swallow, you might find you get an upset stomach and it's certainly not for everyone.

You need to make yourself mentally ready before lucid dreaming and before taking galantamine. The best way to do this is by performing certain exercises.

For example, you shouldn't try to lucid dream after having a few drinks or after a horror movie. Instead, do something that will help you relax and place you in a state of calm such as listening to soothing music.

The best way to use galantamine is via a strategy commonly referred to as wake-back-to-bed WBTB.

Here, you simply sleep for between 4 to 5 hours, wake up, then fall back asleep again. There are two main benefits of this method. First, in case you are having nightmares, you can cut them short. Secondly, you increase the odds of having lucid dreams.

So how do you use the WBTB method?

Start by setting an alarm before you go to bed. It should wake you up 4 or 5 hours into your sleep. Take galantamine then go back to sleep.

It doesn't really have to be any more complicated than that. Take the supplement as soon as you wake up after 5 hours of sleep. Once yo've taken it, lay back down and go back to sleep. As you fall asleep, REALLY set your intention of lucid dreaming.

Think about it as much as you possibly can. You might find it useful to do the 'staircase' technique. Imagine yourself walking down a set of stairs (or walking up). Count in your head each step, and after each step say 'I'm lucid' in your head.

So as you walk down, you'd say 1, I'm lucid, 2, I'm lucid, and so on. Keep going until you reach 500 or so.

What you'll find is that you'll become lucid WAY before you reach 500 if you're dong it slowly. You'll be surprised at just how fast you become lucid actually, especially because you've just taken galantamine and it's the PERFECT time of the night to lucid dream.

Note that for first time users, you will need to begin with a small dose of 4 milligrams. This will likely be a single tablet.

The effects of galantamine will not be immediate however. It will take a complete hour for the drug to be broken down and reach your brain. Keep in mind that using galantamine does not guarantee that you will achieve lucid dreaming.

However, your odds are greatly improved. In case you fail to lucid dream on the first try, continue until you are successful. When the dreams finally do come, you will find that they will be consistent from then on as well as INTENSE.

A study done by Stephen LaBerge has shown that galantamine, when used correctly can increase the chances of lucid dreaming by up to 5 times.

Huperzine-A: The classic lucid pill

This is one of the most well known herbs or supplements used for lucid dreams. This herb has been used for centuries in Asia; however, it has only become more popular in the West as an aid for lucid dreaming in recent years.

It serves as an acetylcholine re-uptake inhibitor and is helpful for being able to access the memory bank while asleep. Research has demonstrated that having access to memory while asleep makes it more likely for lucid dreams auto happen.

What this means is that it prevents acetylcholine being broken down and expiring. Imagine that the more acetylcholine we have in our system, the sharper our memories and critical functions are.

In a normal brain, we slowly lose acetylcholine over time so that the levels remain constant.

By PREVENTING acetylcholine being broken down by the body we can increase the amount of it in our system, meaning we increase our mental sharpness.

This means lucid dreaming is more likely, and we're more likely to remember detailed and vivid dreams.

Huperzine A is also found in Claridream because it makes dreams so vivid and intense. It's so strong that it's measured in tiny measurements (millionths of a gram) and should only really be used once or twice a week at most.

In a nutshell, remember at the start of this book when we spoke about how acetylcholine is essential for memory and dreaming? Well, Huperzine A lets us create and keep MORE of that in our bodies.

It's a great supplement and one you can take at any time of the night, even just as you're going to sleep. Just like most supplements however, they have a half life. There is a perfect time to take them and for most people that IS about 3 hours before you naturally wake up.

There aren't really many side effects, although every substance has side effects for certain people. It's a fairly mild supplement and one you can experiment with quite easily.

Important note: Some people have actually found that Huperzine A LIMITS their ability to remember dreams and makes it harder to become lucid.

This is something you'll have to experiment with yourself.

There isn't much research into this and so most of the reports about Huperzein A are subjective. I'd say one thing could be happening is that Huperzine A could be creating a REM rebound effect, meaning it makes yo more likely to be lucid later on.

If that's the case, experiment with taking it EARLIER in the night, for example as soon as you go to sleep. This will answer that question!

I've had success with both methods but that might just be because I can ALREADY naturally lucid dream, so it's hard to say which supplement had which effect.

Calea Zacatechichi: The dream herb

Calea Zacatechichi improves vivid images in dreams and it also increases the likelihood of lucid dreams. It is native to Mexico and has long been known for its effect on the dreaming life.

It's been used by the Chontal Indians as a tool for dream divination for many centuries. Chontal shamans frequently smoke a cigarette and drink tea made of Calea Zacatechichi before going to sleep. Dreams inspired by this herb give them the answers they are seeking for pressing questions.

Often called the "dream herb," Calea zacatechichi has become more well known outside of its use by the Chontal. Calea zacatechichi is said to cause an increase in the following:

- Frequency of lucid dreams experienced

- Recall ability

- Strength of hypnagogic imagery

- Greater likelihood of spontaneous lucid dream experiences

- More clarity and realism in dreams

If you take this when you're awake, there aren't really any effects that you'll notice, other than maybe feeling a bit more relaxed, tired, and sometimes if you close your eyes you'll notice a few hypnagogic imagery on your eyelids as you would if you were trying to go to sleep.

The best way I'd suggest starting out with this, is to take some of the tincture after about 6 hours of sleep.

You COULD take it right before bed but the effects might not be as potent. It's best to take it JUST before or during your REM sleep in the early morning!

You could certainly combine this with the CAT technique (Cycle adjustment technique) for some great results!

One of the most common ways of taking the dream herb is just by smoking the leaves in a standard roll up cigarette. Just like you'd roll up tobacco and smoke it, or cannabis (if that's your thing) you can use the dried leaves of calea, and smoke them.

People have reported that is the easiest or best way to take it but sometimes the smoke can be quite harsh, depending on the quality of the leaves and how well you roll it, what filter you use and other things. Just be careful.

It might be worth investing in a small water filtered bong if you're planing on smoking this, so you can filter and cool the smoke before inhaling it. This is the best way of ingesting it and getting the substance to directly enter your bloodstream.

Lots of people who take calea zacatechichi say it's easier to just grow the leaves yourself, and then use them in a tea, or smoke them. This saves buying the leaves again and again and waiting for them to arrive, and it's like a little ritual you can perform.

Having the plant in your room can make it feel more special and adventurous, as it's like you're part of the growing process and see the leaves from start to finish as they enter your bloodstream. You can get the seeds here and it's easy to grow them!

Another way of ingesting calea zacatechichi is swallowing a pill or capsule. This means no waiting to tea to boil, no rolling up the leaves and having to go outside to smoke them (or inside if you smoke inside), just pop a pill and go to sleep. You can get those fairly easily.

Brewing the leaves into a tea can taste really bad, but can be effective for getting the active ingredients into your system. Despite how bad it tastes, if you can get used to it or counteract the bad taste somehow, it's a relaxing way of taking it!

Everyone likes a relaxing cup of tea every now and then, and so if you can stomach the bad taste, this could be a good way for you to take it. Just brew the leaves into boiling water and then filter out the leaves as you would with teabagless tea.

A great way to counter act the bitterness of the tea is to suck a sweet while drinking it, or eat a couple of strong mints before drinking it so your taste buds are slightly numbed and have the minty taste on them.

Mixing dream herb with cannabis has been said to sort of supplement the effects and make things seem that bit less negative. The combination has been said to make you more relaxed, and after a while, even has mild hallucinogenic effects.

It's also said that mixing strong weed and calea z can make things a little bit hazy. Maybe this is because the effects sort of cancel each other out and make your vision and thinking blurry.

Mixing dream herb with Mugwort has some surprising effects. Because you can already get dream support and an increase in vividness from EITHER of these two leaves/herbs, mixing them can boost this effect.

In fact, mixing different types of dream inducing herbs is not a new idea. Mixing natural dream supporting herbs can sometimes boost the effect of both. It's a case of 1 plus 1 making 3.

Calea zacatechichi can be a bit rough if you're not used to it or expecting it. Just be prepared that you MIGHT throw up at first, and you might feel dizzy and need to sit down. These effects usually pass and so after that, it's not really dangerous at all.

Much like cannabis, you can just stop when you feel you've had enough, and even then, calea z effects are so mild that you probably will just go to sleep and have some nice dreams!

Blue Lotus

Blue Lotus is a subtle herb and its effects are not as strong as you might expect.

Blue Lotus gives a gentle sense of tranquillity and euphoria and also provides an altered sense of consciousness. Using Blue Lotus will enhance meditative and introspective practices.

There is also often a feeling of warmth around the head and upper body and a floating feeling reported while under the influence of Blue Lotus. Many users reports an increase in lucidity after ingesting this herb.

The Blue Lotus is typically taken as a tea, with a recommended dose of 5 grams per person, steeped in boiling water and then allowed to cool before drinking it directly. The Egyptians also used to soak it in wine for hours at a time, at the same dose of 5 grams per bottle.

In its guise as an oil concentrate, the Blue Lotus plant is a very effective sedative. In fact, the absolute oil of this plant is so potent that just massaging it into the skin can instantly absorb the alkaloids, which then induces the effects that it's so famous for.

Just be sure not to confuse the absolute oil concentrate with the essential oil, as the latter is made through steam distillation and has a reduced overall potency. Nevertheless, it is still a viable method of consuming the plant and producing the desired effects.

That said the psychoactive effects of the plant are specifically found in the buds and flowers, which are then compressed into a sticky resin to make a hash-like substance that you can smoke, while a Blue Lotus tincture is available if you prefer that method.

You can also drink the plant as a tea, made by steeping it into boiling water and then allowing it to cool while absorbing all the aromas and activating its constituents for maximum effect, and soaking it in wine for several hours will also have the same result.

As you can see, there is an endless array of options to choose from when it comes to consuming the plant. You can smoke it, drink it as a tea, wine, or massage it onto your skin as an absolute or essential oil. Now let's take a look at its effects to see what the after effects of consuming it are.

Blue lotus side effects

The Blue Lotus is quite tame when compared to other popular lucid dreaming aids, but it makes for an ideal plant to use for newbies. Its effects typically kick in within the first half an hour after use, and usually start out as a mild stimulant with a slight tingling sensation throughout the body.

The plant is also characterised by a heightened awareness, mental clarity, and a sense of serenity coupled with unparalleled euphoria.

It's also known as an aphrodisiac as it enhances tactile senses, and has worked really well for sufferers of erectile dysfunction that's brought on by depression. It can also be extremely calming, while producing uniquely detailed dreams with enhanced colors and vivid detail.

For those who want to enter a meditative state, then taking the plant as a tea is your best bet, while pairing it with wine works great when you just want to explore its awareness amplifying qualities and create a lively vibe during social interactions.

The actual dream trip of the Blue Lotus plant can only be described as unique, and usually starts while you're still awake, and then seamlessly transitions to the dream state.

It almost feels as though the dream state and the waking state blend into one and you're able to experience life with penetrating sensitivity. Apart from its psychedelic qualities, the Blue Lotus is lauded for its healing abilities as well, and is widely used as a sleep aid and natural stress reliever.

In addition, certain studies have shown that the Blue Lotus plant works really well to treat gastrointestinal problems, particularly diarrhoea and dyspepsia.

The Blue Lotus has travelled across centuries and borders, spreading its fragrant aroma and unique healing abilities for all to enjoy, and today we have the full benefit of understanding and purposefully utilising these abilities.

While it may not be in the TOP tier of lucid dreaming aids, it is still a viable healing herb to use when experiencing any form of stress and/or depression. Hopefully it'll be legalised in the countries where it has been banned, because it is a mild plant with no seriously adverse side effects.

To be completely honest, Blue Lotus doesn't have a huge effect on lucid dreams. It does improve them but nowhere near as much as some of the other supplements mentioned in this book or online. It's still cheap and easy to buy in most places though, so worth a look!

Mugwort: The herb of lucidity

Mugwort is a herb that is frequently used for assistance in lucid dreaming. It can be used to make a "dream pillow" and can be used in tea or capsule form.

It is an attractive option because it is one of the least expensive dream herbs. Dream pillows are a powerful way of using herbs like mugwort to make it easier to fall asleep, and easier to dream lucidly. While not considered the most powerful herb for lucid dreams, it's still a useful herb for boosting dreams.

The suggested dosage varies from person to person so make sure you research it and consult a doctor first. The suggested daily dosage of mugwort for lucid dreaming, is about 150mg. A word of warning though, it can leave you feeling quite dehydrated so make sure to drink enough water during the day!

4 Ways of taking Mugwort

Here are the most common methods for ingesting mugwort. You'll find that one or two will stand out to you as the better choices. For example, if you don't smoke, this is not an option. If you don't like tea or drinking hot beverages, that's not an option etc...

1: Smoking It

Not a great one if you're not a smoker, but it's common to smoke the leaves. You can roll it up in a rolling paper just like you would a normal cigarette. It can also be mixed with tobacco, or you could go for the traditional 'sailor' method and use it instead of tobacco!

2: A Mugwort Dream Pillow

A very popular way to use Mugwort is to make a dream pillow. This means putting a few leaves or incense inside your pillow case. The aroma will enter your system and help you become lucid. You can mix it with another incense or herb, like Lavender. Making a dream pillow is a great way to have restful nights and increase the chances of becoming lucid!

3: Burning The Incense

The incense of Mugwort can be burned to stimulate dreams and relax you. This is probably the least common method but it's worth a try! I'd suggest trying several methods of consumption and seeing which one has the best result!

4: Drinking Mugwort Tea

One of the most common ways to consume Mugwort is to *brew the leaves into a tea*. This can be the easiest way as well. Non smokers commonly use this method combined with making a Mugwort dream pillow.

To make a tea, prepare the leaves by bushing off any dirt and soil. Then add one teaspoon of the leaves (roughly) to the teapot. Filter it and then drink!

Don't take if pregnant!

***If you're pregnant, or think you're pregnant, DO NOT
USE MUGWORT.***

It stimulates menstruation, and it's been said to induce a period in women.

Some people use it to ease the passing of their 'time of the month' so don't use it if you even think you're pregnant.

Choline bitartrate: Dream memory juice

Choline bitartrate can improve dream recall; however, it has other benefits as well. It is considered to be a memory boosting supplement that also has ability to improve lucid dreaming.

Choline bitartrate supplements have Nootropic (brain enhancing) effects including cognitive improvements as well as mental stimulation. It is also an anti-inflammatory remedy and has powerful benefits for the heart.

It's is actually found in the body in small amounts and is involved with maintaining and supporting mental function. It supports cognitive ability, memory and focus. (Essential for lucid dreaming, right?).

The body only produces a small amount and therefore it's important to get the rest from a healthy diet. Here are some foods that contain small amounts of Choline:

- Brussel sprouts

- Peanuts

- Broccoli

So it's likely that you already consume some amount of Choline. Why am I referencing it only as Choline regarding the food you eat?

Because usually it is just 'Choline' and then when it's used as a supplement it's combined with a salt such as 'Bitartrate'.

Therefore, Choline Bitartrate refers to just the supplement form, and negates the fact you can actually get it from diet as well.

Nevertheless, it's great to get it in supplement form as well, as this gives a more powerful does and you'll experience the effects more. You'll notice an improvement in mental clarity, memory, focus and cognitive processing abilities. You'll just 'think' better.

The suggested dosage for Choline Bitartrate (for lucid dreaming at least) is about 650mg, rising up to 2g in the case of some men, but somewhere between those two lies the average recommended dose.

Anything above that could be considered dangerous, and shouldn't be attempted. For best results, we'd say take 800mg daily as well as a healthy diet including Choline as well.

So it's obvious that Choline has a positive impact on your dream life and the way you are mentally 'present' in a lucid dream.

Here's how you can use it to have deeper and more vivid lucid dreams. Here's the best way to use choline to have better lucid dreams:

- Make sure you're writing your dreams down. In your dream journal, after each night of dreams, write how much choline you took the night before, and what techniques (if any) you used

- You might find that a smaller dose works better for you than a larger dose, experiment!

- Try one of the following techniques combined with taking choline either just before bed, or AS you're doing the technique

- Remember that it's always best to experiment with yourself. You might find that it works best when mixed with dream tea or something like vitamin B6. Test test test!

DreamLeaf: Enter the Matrix

These pills are said to be modeled on the movie "The Matrix." This is because one is red and one's blue. It's a very nice look and helps get you into the mindset of 'I'm going to take this and lucid dream'.

It is considered to be a very good choice for beginner lucid dreamers. It's taken in two parts and one pill is taken before going to sleep and the other is taken after 4-5 hours of sleep.

Users of the DreamLeaf supplement report a strong increase in lucidity, but don't expect instant results.

As with all dream supplements, it's important to use dream induction techniques in addition to supplements. Supplements alone will not achieve the desired results.

The way it actually works is by using the two pills to target different parts of your sleep. The blue pill taken at the start of the night contains things like Mugwort and Valerian root which help you fall asleep faster.

They also promote memory and relaxation but mainly they're just to get you to fall asleep quickly and deeply.

Then the red pill is taken later on in the night after you've slept for 4-5 hours. You an see a trend here towards taking supplements during the night after 4-5 hours of sleep, because it works the best that way.

The ideal solution would be a pill that ONLY releases it's active ingredients at that time, meaning you don't have to wake yourself up at all, you just take a pill and experience an entire nights sleep and dreams.

But that's not real just yet! So DreamLeaf targets your REM sleep during the early hours of the morning with the red pill. The red pill contains things like Huperzine Z, Alpha GPC and Choline. It's a pretty good way of lucid dreaming if you're new, and there's a lot of science behind the ingredients and how they work.

Ginkgo Biloba (memory and blood flow)

Ginkgo Biloba is a well known supplement on the market that improves memory and brain function. Because it boosts memory and cognitive speed, it will likely lead to better dreams. Ginkgo Biloba has been used by the Chinese for these purposes for centuries.

How does it work? It mainly improves blood flow to the brain which boosts cognitive function and speed as well as critical thinking skills. Because of these qualities, it's also used as a treatment for Alzheimers.

Lots of supplements that ONLY increase blood flow to the brain actually cause people to have more vivid dreams as a side effect, so there's something to be said about things that can do that.

It's not a direct effect, but it's certainly something you'll notice if you take it. Gingko is actually an ingredient in many nootropics, and not always for it's dream enhancing abilities.

I've tried this one with great success for dream RECALL, but I can't say it made me any more lucid. It's something again that's easy to get online and well worth experimenting with.

Heimia Salicifolia: The Sun opener

Heima Salicifolia (also called the sun opener) is an herb that can be used to summon 'life altering' dreams. Used by the ancient ancient Aztecs, the sun opener is said to allow the user to retrieve distant memories that they do not remember in waking life.

It's also said to bring advanced hearing abilities. Users say they are able to hear far away sounds when taking Heimia and that this effect can last for several hours. It's also sometimes called the "Elixir of the Sun."

It is a particular favorite of Mexican shamans, and they have used the flowers in ceremonies for centuries.

Many of them also refer to the flower, which grow up to 1.5 meters, as sinicuici—

which refers to its auditory hallucinogenic qualities.

The plant itself is very common looking and at first glance offers no indication of its supernatural power—with its thin branches and yellow flowers that are about two centimeters in width.

The traditional method of using Heimia Salicifolia was to allow the yellow flowers to completely wilt and dry, and then add cool water to them in a jar or container.

Allowing the dried flowers to ferment for 24 hours is necessary for maximum effect. Shamans believe that the power of Heimia Salicifolia is infused through the sun during the fermentation process. Because of this, some refer to it as the "elixir of the sun."

After fermentation happens, the mixture is strained and put in a tea. At least a third of an ounce is used, but many say that at least half an ounce is needed for a deeper experience. The main ingredient is phenylalanine which mimics the effects of dopamine and adrenaline—which, of course, accounts for its pleasurable effect.

With minimal to moderate use, most do not experience any substantial side effects. Heimia Salicifolia does not seem to affect energy levels after use. However, the yellow tint in vision may last for more time than expected.

Some report that this side effect can last up to a day after using the herb. Not many people use the "Sun Opener" on a long-term basis but if that is done, there may be long-term effects.

This is a substance that's a lot harder to research and buy than most others. If you find a way of getting it, make sure you research it and try only the smallest dose at first. There are many other supplements that are a lot easier to use and find!

Wild Asparagus Root

Also called the "flying herb" because of its ability to produce that feeling while sleeping, wild asparagus is said to open up the heart and improve its energy.

The Chinese word for wild asparagus root is "Tian Men Dong" which translates to "heavenly spirit herb." For centuries, it's been used by shamans, monks, and yogis for its effects on consciousness.

The best way to use wild asparagus is to brew a tea from the root. A tea from the fresh root will be much more potent than a tea brewed from a drier root. Then filter it to remove all the remnants. Drink it quickly and then attempt to go to sleep.

Valerian root (memory booster)

Valerian is well known for its ability to induce sleep and help people fall asleep faster. It is also used to induce profound lucid dreams as well.

An added benefit is that it also treats joint pain and headaches and depression. It's a sedative and relaxant making it useful for falling asleep faster and deeper.

Valerian also improves dream recall which is the first step in achieving lucidity in dreams.

Once you are able to remember your dreams regularly, it's possible to become conscious while in the dream state. Valerian's ability to make our dreams more vivid is one of the reasons it is easier to remember dreams while taking Valerian.

The stranger our dreams become, the easier it is to realize we are dreaming, which of course makes it much easier to achieve lucidity.

While Valerian is effective in aiding dream recall, it is best taken in addition to other more potent dream herbs.

Although it is a Western herb, Valerian root has a long history of use in Traditional Chinese Medicine (TCM) and is one of the most prevalent non-Chinese herbs used in TCM.

Valerian root was bought to China by western traders and has since been included in the TCM materia medica.

While western practitioners tend to prescribe Valerian root as a sleep aid, in China it is considered to be a spirit-quieting medicine with a blood moving action.

Its nature and flavour are documented as being acrid, sweet and warm and its channel energies are the heart and liver.

It is used to nourish the heart, quiet the spirit, alleviate insomnia. It is viewed as a heart-opening and heart nourishing herb that is used in tandem with other herbs that quiet the mind and focus one's attention on the heart centre.

It is also used to treat menstrual problems, amenorrhea, swelling and generalised body pains.

The reason that the Chinese were so ready to adopt Valerian into their medicinal system is because of the belief that Kuan Yin resides in this herb. Kuan (earth) Yin (the spiritual energy that ebbs and flows).

The spiritual properties attributed to Valerian are gentle healing powers, reconciliation between loved ones, promoting feelings of love and devotion and easing pain and loneliness. Valerian profoundly improves dream recall, which, as any lucid dreamer knows, is the first step we need to take in achieving lucidity in dreams.

Once you are able to remember your dreams on a daily basis, you are able to go one step further by becoming conscious while you are in the dream state.

Valerian's ability to make our dreams more vivid (and more bizarre!) is one of the reasons it is easier to recall dreams when we work with Valerian. The wackier our dreams, the easier it is to realise we are dreaming, which makes it much easier to have a lucid dream.

It should be noted that while Valerian is great at aiding in dream recall and enhancing dream content (i.e. making dreams vivid and strange), it is best taken in tandem with other more powerful dream herbs.

It is important to understand the role of active ingredients when we think about taking a dream herb.

For example, the active ingredient in Valerian is valerenic acid and when we are looking to promote dream recall we can choose to either supplement with "straight" Valerian or with a special dream mixture that contains Valerian along with other plants.

If you want to take pure Valerian, you are going to have to take a relatively high dose and so it is important to look for a supplement that contains at least 450-600mg of valerenic acid for it to be effective.

If taking Valerian liquid extract, look for a brand that boasts 4:1 strength ratio (a valerenic content of around 0.8%).

Peppermint

Peppermint is known to support dream quality and often makes dream scenes more vivid and engaging. Peppermint can be ingested by tincture or in tea. Many people drink this in a tea because it tastes better than other dream herbs.

Another way to benefit from peppermint is to soak in a bath with some peppermint oil infused into the bath water before bed. Not only will your dreams become more vivid, you will feel relaxed and refreshed from the effects of the peppermint oil.

Make sure to research this one and check it against anything you're currently already taking. There have been reports of peppermint interfering with some things and substances, causing issues. For most of us it's a fairly mild effect, and doesn't really cause too much trouble but if you're already on medications, it can make them less effective.

What I would say with this one is to not think of it as a supplement. Think of the essential oil as a relaxation aid that you can add to your bath, or put under your pillow.

The best results I've had from peppermint were to add a few drops of the essential oil to my dream pillow. I also got some relaxed dreams by soaking in a bath with 1 parts peppermint essential oil to 2 parts lavender essential oil in the bath. I think I used about 6-10 drops in total.

Silene Capensis

Silene Capensis is a oneirongen commonly used in South Africa. It is often associated with the Xhosa tribe and they have long used it to bring powerful dreams. Silence capensis help with dream recall so powerfully, that even a small amount will help the user remember dreams in GREAT detail the next morning.

What is the best way to take this herb?

Its recommended to use the powdered form to make a strong tea and then filter and drink. It's best to drink first thing in the morning because it takes a while to take effect. It's not recommended to take before bed because the effects won't be as powerful.

Don't use too much the first time. 200 mg is more than enough to start because larger doses can actually cause some people to throw up. For this reason, it's often used as a cleansing herb in some tribes.

The roots of the flowering Silene Capensis plant contain psychoactive components which have earned it a status as an 'AChEI inhibitor', meaning that it's an effective lucid dreaming aid.

You can tell just from the robust aroma emitted by this plant, that it's a truly entrancing herb.

For ages the Xhosa shaman of South Africa have widely used the plant to experience richly intense and clear dreams, and subsequently gave it the name 'undlela zimhlophe' or white paths due to its ability to connect them with the ancestors, which they also refer to as 'white spirits'.

The Xhosa peoples revere the Silene Capensis plant as a powerful and sacrosanct healing herb, and while some take it for its purgative effects that cleanse mind, body and spirit, it mostly shines as a ceremonial plant.

For example, during the Xhosa traditional death ceremony, the plant is used to bring closure and peace between the departed and the living, while it is also used in the Xhosa culture's shaman initiation ceremony, where inductees undergo a 3-day full moon excursion, sans meat, sex and alcohol.

This 3-day session usually occurs at a secluded location, so that initiates can fully benefit from the potent effects of the Silene Capensis root, the object of which is to experience intensely symbolic dreams.

When taking the plant for lucid dreaming purposes, it's important to remember to use the roots, as that's where the psychoactive components are.

You can purchase the root from a reputable online vendor, where it will most likely be referred to as 'Silene Capensis Whole Root'.

The root is primed by first breaking it up into tiny pieces, after which you steep it in cold water and store it in the fridge overnight. Or you can purchase an already powdered root which you'll then steep in cold water over night, using a ratio of 1 teaspoon of powder to 2 cups of water.

All you have to do the following morning is to shake the bottle up until a full-bodied white froth forms, or stir it with a fork until you see the froth forming, and then drink it straight up until you're so full that you feel like vomiting.

This is actually a good thing, because you're required to do a bit of voluntary purging through vomiting, as one would do when using ayahuasca, in order to prepare your system for what's to come.

For some, it usually takes several hours before the effects start to kick in, and if you want you can consume breakfast at least an hour after taking the root to keep your strength up, although that's entirely up to you.

Others will require a few more doses in order to feel the effects and if that's the case with you then you can feel free to drink it in the morning and the evening as well.

It's also a good idea to have someone with you during the trip, especially if it's your first time experimenting with lucid dreaming herbs, but if you're a pro then you probably already know what to do.

There are other methods of taking Selene Capensis that you could try such as chewing the roots or drinking it as a tea, where you'd stir the powdered roots into boiling water and then drink it after it's cooled down.

Another nice one to try, would be to wash oneself with the frothy mixture, a practice which forms part of the Xhosa initiation ceremony, and is said to have purging effects that enhance the quality of the subsequent dream state.

Although there is no reported dosage limit for the Silene Capensis root, it's probably wise to take the recommended dose of 1 heaped teaspoon of powdered root to 2 cups of water, once or twice per day until you experience the desired outcome.

While most people experience the effects of the root within hours of taking it, others require a few more doses over the course of a few days before they experience anything at all.

This might explain why Xhosa shaman initiates take the root over the course of 3 days in order to experience its full effects.

Just be sure to apply the golden rule, which is to use caution and moderation and as with any lucid dream herb, never use it for more than a week without taking a break.

It's important to keep in mind as you explore the possibilities presented by the Silene Capensis root that your experiences may vary from those reported by the native Xhosa shamans.

Suppliers also differ in the quality that they provide, and while some provide the real thing, others sell a watered-down version that leaves much to be desired.

Also, you might have to tinker with the dosage a bit before you get the right amount that's able to induce the experiences that this root is so famous for.

Mullein

No list is complete without at least one herb that is used primarily as protection on the dreamscape. Mullein is said to ward off nightmares while sleeping. It's been commonly used by tribes for millennia to have less frightening dreams.

It also helps one fall asleep when ingested, and it makes an excellent tea for bringing prophetic dreams. Some recommend keeping Mullein leaves under the pillow to ward off bad dreams.

Important WARNING
about any supplements

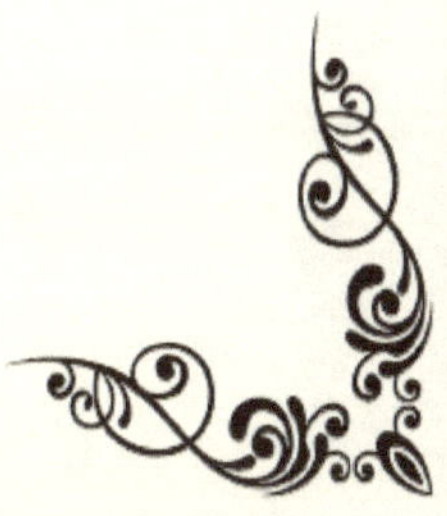

Important warnings about ANY supplements

We need to mention some warnings about supplements that you NEED to listen to before trying anything.

Don't combine different lucid dream supplements unless you are sure you know what you're doing.

Consulting with professionals is always recommended in order to prevent poor reactions with other medications and supplements.

If you are pregnant or have other significant medical issues, always be sure to take the proper precautions. Taking multiple drugs/ supplements at the same time can be very dangerous.

As with anything taken on a regular basis, it's possible to build up a tolerance to dream supplements. This means that the more you use something, the more you HAVE to use to get the same effect.

There are some supplements however which have the reverse effect. The more of them you use, the more strong and potent the effects get.

This means you CONSTANTLY need to check the dosages of everything you're taking, and make sure you know what you're doing to stay safe.

For best results, vary supplements taken in order to prevent this from happening and to discover which ones work best for you.

If you notice decreased results with a supplement after using it for a period of time, try taking a break and "cycling"

them to help combat increased tolerance
to a particular supplement.

SUPPLEMENTS *and* TECHNIQUES:
Using *them in tandem*

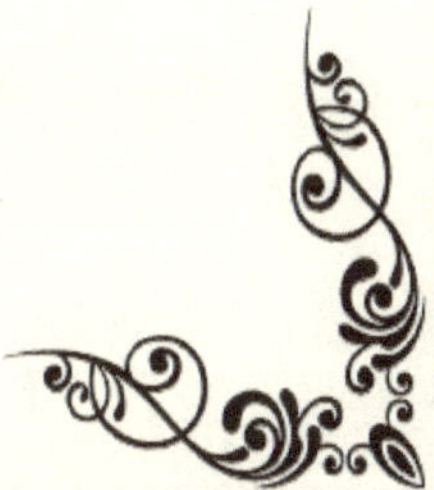

Using induction techniques in tandem with supplements

We've spoken in detail about various types of supplements and how they work on the body, but we need to talk about how to use them in combination with actual lucid dreaming techniques.

This means you're going to need to make notes for this section, (or just refer back to this while you're trying the methods).

The RAUSIS Technique

Jean Rausis developed a technique called, appropriately enough, the Rausis method for lucid dreaming. The Swiss researcher has a lot of experience in manipulating the conscious state of the mind in order to gain lucidity. The Rausis technique is said to be very accessible for beginners to be able to have lucid dreams even on the first attempt.

The method is very straightforward. Perhaps you can remember a time when an external noise was included in a dream?

This ability of the brain to incorporate a sound into a dream is what is being used in this technique.

Basically, when the body hears a noise in real life, the mind will incorporate that noise into the dream to try to make sense of it. People who use this technique sometimes set an alarm or have someone call them during REM sleep to achieve this effect.

I won't go into detail on the technique but I would suggest trying this with memory or vividness enchanting supplements. Try this technique in combination with **Claridream** to make the dreams more vivid and intense.

Reality checks with supplements

This is probably the most well-known lucid dreaming exercise. Reality checks are the secret weapon of those who tend towards spontaneous lucid dreams. In essence, when you're dreaming you begin realize you're dreaming and then lucidity happens.

When doing a reality check, attempt an impossible action in the waking world (such as placing your hand through a wall) while asking yourself if you are dreaming or not. Here's an example of a reality check:

The finger palm push: In real life, you will always get the same response and the same feeling, the resistance, the tension and the feeling of your finger pressing your palm will be constant.

In the dream however, the finger will go through your palm, and you likely won't feel it either. It will certainly feel strange, and you'll realise that something's not right, therefore allowing you to become Lucid.

Reality checks are used to discern whether you're dreaming or not. When awake, it's a way of creating a habit. The effects of asking yourself throughout the day if you're awake or not make their way into your dreams.

This is the purpose of a reality check— to get to the point of having the mind trained to ask if something is real or not in a dream.

Strive to do 10-20 reality checks randomly throughout your day. Consider wearing a digital watch and perform a reality check every time it chimes. This programs the question into your mind and before long you'll spontaneously perform a reality check in a dream. When this happens, it won't be long before you're lucid!

When you first wake up in the morning is the best time to do a reality check. Doing this will probably save you lots of frustration and will prevent false awakenings.

Doing this will eventually ensure that you don't have false awakenings which will, in turn, lead to more lucid dreams.

If you are prone to having recurring dreams, use this as a tool to figure out when you're dreaming. The first step is to familiarize yourself fully with your recurring dream by writing about it in a dream journal.

Once you've written out the dream, read every detail of the dream repeatedly until you know the dream with great specificity. Each night as you go to bed, read your dream story and set your intentions to become lucid. When you have the recurring dream, you will recognize it and have a much greater chance of becoming lucid.

Wake Induced Lucid Dream (WILD) & Huperzine A

The basics of this technique are to stay focused and keep concentrating on staying awake while letting the body go into sleep paralysis.

This allows you to skip reality checks because you don't go to sleep the first place—or at least you don't in the mind. Your body goes to sleep though and becomes unable to move. The muscles become paralyzed and your body temperature will decrease.

You are basically sleeping, but you are able to stay awake in the dream—which leads to a lucid dream. It's an effective technique because it promotes relaxation and meditation before sleeping which increases overall health.

Step 1: Lay down and get comfortable

Lay down in your bed, scratch any itches you have, make sure your muscles are stretched out, you have yawned, sorted your pillows out etc, anything you need to do in order to go to sleep, do this now.

It's important because the following steps require you to not move at all! If you move past this point you'll have to start again.

This is the time also to finally check your room, and ensure lights are all off, nothing is plugged in or making a light/

noise. You're comfortable and relaxed. Try and suppress any thoughts you are having, any worries or memories, just observe them, and let them slip away.

Don't interact with them, or think about them such as what you'll do tomorrow, just observe the thoughts, and let them drift away. Think of nothing. It might help to improve your sleep conditions by getting some incense or a decent mattress.

Step 2: The relaxation stage

Now you focus on your muscles. Feel the tension and let it go. Relax every single part of your body, do it in sections and move all along your body so that every muscle is relaxed, start at your feet, then up through your legs, back, chest, arms, neck and face.

There is a lot of tension held in the jaw and the face which is usually unnoticed, but it's there. focus on your face and jaw more than the rest of your body, and let go of the tension. You should be completely relaxed and limp, supported only by your mattress.

Step 3: Control your breathing

Now that your muscles are relaxed, you can focus on your breathing, feel the breath go into your mouth and out through your nose, or whichever way is the most comfortable, but make sure you're breathing deeply and in a fashion which doesn't make you uncomfortable.

As you're laying there, feel your heartbeat. Not with your hands on your chest, but rather just try and feel it beating through your chest. You can feel it if you pay attention.

Now try to lower it. This is something which takes practice, so if you can't lower your heartbeat just by laying there, just move on to the next step. If you are able to do this, lower it to a relaxed rate.

Step 4: Try to visualise and hear sounds

Spend about 10-20 minutes on the last step, making sure you're totally relaxed and comfortable. This is important for the later stages.

Now you're going to try and 'see' images and shapes. Your eyes are closed, and you're relaxed but you're going to visualise things.

Start by imagining a circle. Just a plain ring in front of you. When you can see that circle, make it clearer. Now make it disappear. Get the circle back, and keep bringing shapes up this way and get good at thinking about a shape and then seeing it in front of you.

Now start playing around with it, make it bigger, change the colour, and make it start to move.

Spin the circle round. Now after a while you'll be able to visualise more complex things, try seeing a beach.

An island in the distance, and you'll find that as you 'go with it' the environment seems to create itself. You need to do less and less, and are now just seeing it create itself.

Decide on a basic setting for the dream, such as a forest or an island, something easy with not a lot of movement, just the waves and the trees swaying in the breeze.

Really visualise it and try to see the details, but focus more on 'seeing' them than imagining them. Think as though the beach is already there, but you just can't see it.

Step 5: Insert yourself into the dream environment

Now you start to put yourself and your awareness into that environment. Start by looking around, turn in a circle in your mind, see what's behind you. Now see if you can look down, do you see your feet? your hands?

Feel the temperature, and listen for the sounds in the background. *What do you feel?* the sand on your bare feet? Tell yourself that you're dreaming, and that it's all in your head. You can now move around, and interact with the world. Your body is asleep but your mind is now creating a world around you.

You're in a lucid dream now!

You've just created your Lucid Dream using the WILD technique! Now you're in the dream, and you're semi-lucid, it's time to start stabilising the dream, maybe do a couple of reality checks, just to make sure, and it's very important at this stage to keep calm, and not run around yelling *'I'm Dreaming'*, that's a classic beginner mistake.

And that's how to perform a Wake initiated lucid dream, or WILD for short. It does take a lot of practice because it's not something you'll be used to and it's a new skill. When you do perfect it, however, it will allow you to directly induce a lucid dream. Some of my best lucid dreams have come from using the WILD technique.

To combine Huperzine A with this technique, perform the technique in the early hours of the morning straight after taking your

Huperzine A supplement. You could use something like Dreamleaf for this.

From my experience, you have to take the supplement without waking yourself up too much. I found it was useful to have everything laid out next to the bed ready to take it, before going back to sleep again.

You might also need a small snack to eat at the same time, to aid digestion and make sure you avoid upset stomach! I find I ALWAYS get sick and nauseous when taking a supplement or pill on an empty stomach.

Visually Incubated Lucid Dream (VILD) and Claridream

A VILD is a lucid dreaming induction technique that involves

practicing a dream scene before actually going to sleep.

The scene you visualize includes a reality check in the scene and should be simple for best results.

The idea is that by visualizing the dream scene during the day and before bed, you're more likely to dream about that scene. By including a reality check in the scene, you're more likely to become lucid.

The visually incubated lucid dream is considered to be a very effective technique. This is because you're preparing for the dream scene making it less likely you will wake up.

In lucid dreams, exploring a scene too quickly can make you wake up or have a blackout. This technique avoids that issue because you already know what the dream scene will be like.

To perform the VILD you need to practice visualising a simple dream scene INVOLVING a reality check. It needs to be easy to see and re-create, and the details should be simple. You can use paradoxes like in Inception if you find that easier.

You include a reality check in the scene by visualising it there. An example could be you visualise a dream scene in which you're on the beach with your friend. You're both looking around at the clouds in the sky, which spell out the words 'Are you dreaming?'.

Notice that the very scene itself IS a reality check, and if you actually dreamed that scene, you'd be very likely to do a reality check, because it's literally spelled out in the clouds you're looking at!

Here's how you do it:

- Keep a dream journal and do 20 reality checks per day

- Design a dream scene and visualise being there several times during the day. Include a reality check in the actual dream scene (The words 'are you dreaming' written on a wall, for example)

- Put a drawing of the dream scene under your pillow and imagine yourself IN the dream

- Create and enter the dream by focusing on it

- Stabilize the dream by spinning round or meditating (while in the lucid dream)

1: Dream journals and reality tests

Like almost any other lucid technique, keeping a dream

journal and doing reality checks are very important. They're the foundations, and can't be ignored.

Many people try and ignore these essentials and then comment on lucid dreaming forums wondering why they can't seem to lucid dream, despite the fact they've read 'every technique out there'. This is why.

To prime yourself for the VILD, simply remember to write your dreams down EVERY morning, in a dream diary. Also, make sure you perform 20 or more reality tests throughout the day.

Once you're sure you've been doing that for about a week or two you can move onto the rest of the VILD method.

2: Designing a dream (With a built in reality check)

Think about what dream scene you want
to visualise and incubate. To start with, it
might be easier to use a beach, forest, city
or something that everyone can easily re-
create in their mind. It's harder to create
and visualise places you've never been to.

So begin painting a mental picture of the
dream scene you're going to incubate,
BUT include a reality check in the scene.

You could imagine yourself on a beach
looking up at clouds that say 'Are you
dreaming?'. Here are some examples of
dream scenes with reality checks built
into them, so you get the idea better:

- You're in your bedroom, looking around
  the walls, but you notice that on all the
  walls in large, red ink are the words
  'You're dreaming'. Everywhere you look,
  this thick, smeared red ink screams
  those words.

- You're on a train, but instead of seats, there are just rows of small beds, each one with what seems to be.. YOU laying down, asleep on them. Dozens of versions of yourself, all sleeping on the train. You hear an announcer shout 'Next station is.. Lucid dreaming. You're in a dream, right now'.

- You're swimming in an ocean of seahorses, and as you look up to the ocean surface, you notice you're breathing underwater. A seahorse turns to you, and says 'you're dreaming'

The reality check needs to be PART of what you're visualising. This makes it more likely to show up in the dream when you actually have it!

Next, draw the dream scene on a piece of paper. It doesn't matter if you're not very good at drawing. Just draw the most simple version of the dream, so that when you look at the drawing you're reminded of the dream scene.

It just needs to nudge you to remember the dream scene. It doesn't need to be a masterpiece. In fact, the more simple the idea, the better it will work! When you've drawn it, fold it up and put it in your pocket.

Every time during the day that you do a reality check, take out the drawing and look at it. As you look as it, imagine yourself actually there, in the dream, tonight.

3: Visualising the dream scene

This step is done when you're going to sleep, so make sure that BEFORE this step, you've gone through your bedtime routine and got ready for bed.

Make sure you're relaxed. It might help to go through some basic relaxation techniques to get ready for sleeping. (If you have trouble falling asleep, check out this soundtrack that helps you fall asleep).

Now, as you're laying in the bed, you must focus on the dream scene. Recall details like what it feels like, what smells, sounds and sights are there.

Use all of your senses to experience the dream. (for those who have TROUBLE visualising things, there's a few tips at the end of this article).

Now, put the drawing you did earlier under your pillow, and tell yourself that you're going to visit that dream right now. I know some of you are thinking that the act of putting it under your pillow won't do anything, but believe me, it does.

It's telling your subconscious mind that the dream is IMPORTANT and needs to be treated with importance. Even if it's just a placebo effect, you should never underestimate the awesome power of the placebo effect.

Now go to sleep, telling yourself that you're going to enter the dream. You can either go to sleep naturally and you should enter the dream directly, and become lucid, OR you can do something else.

Another way of doing it would be to enter the dream using the WBTB method. This involves just setting an alarm and then when you wake up (2 hours before you'd NORMALLY wake up) you visualise the dream scene THEN instead of before going to bed.

4: Creating and entering the dream

Now, you'll naturally have a dream about the dream scene you visualised before. (this works 80% of the time). Because the dream scene you imagined actually included a reality check, you should become naturally lucid at some point.

Want to know the best part? Because you've practiced the lucid dream, you shouldn't actually need to do much from there. You're likely to have the dream you practiced, and it's likely to be STABLE because you've already visualised it, so it won't fade to black!

You can stabilise it even further, if you want:

5: Stabilising the dream when you're in it

You can now stabilise the lucid dream even further by spinning round, or doing some simple maths problems. You shouldn't need to do much at this stage, because you're already used to the scene and it shouldn't blackout!

Another thing: If you want to stay in the VILD for longer, make sure you stay sort of near the starting point. The original dream scene you visualised is the most stable area of the dream. Venturing too far outside of that will make it more likely that you'll wake up.

Mix this technique with the supplement Claridream for a very intense and vivid experience.

Claridream PRO is a great dream enhancer for more vivid and visual dreams. That's why I'd suggest mixing it with the VILD, because it's such a visual technique.

I found that my dreams were about 30-50% more vivid and colourful

when I tried Claridream PRO, and I use it fairly often now for more vivid and intense dreams.

Senses Initiated Lucid Dream (SSILD) and Valerian Root

The SSILD technique is a hybrid lucid dreaming technique which combines several different techniques. How does it work? It works by making the mind focus specifically on your surroundings so that when you fall asleep you're more likely to have a lucid dream.

This combined with the fact that you're doing it at a time when REM sleep is strongest usually means it has a strong chance of working. It's not as vague as some other techniques. It's also very clear and to the point which will please the more practical types among us.

Use Valerian root with this technique to make the falling asleep stage faster. Valerian root has been shown to make falling asleep faster and easier, and it also makes your sleep deeper and more intense.

So it's a great way of having more advanced dream scenes and essentially sedating yourself to stabilise the dream. I've had great results from this and I find that Mugwort and valerian in particular are great at providing this sedation and relaxation in the early stages of sleep.

Interestingly, Mugwort and Valerian are both ingredients in Dream Leafs first pill, the blue pill!

It can work really well to take DreamLeafs blue pill as you fall asleep, and then try the SSILD technique in the later part of the night when you take the red pill. This gives your body and mind all the support it needs to create a lucid dream.

Finger Induced Lucid Dream (FILD) and Gingko Biloba

The FILD technique is a really interesting thing you can do to make yourself lucid in just a few seconds!

The first step is to allow yourself to become really tired. Then lift your middle and index finger up and down like you're playing a piano and playing two notes one after the other quickly, but never both at the same time.

Press them just hard enough so that they press down some, but not all the way down. Now press even lighter than that so you're barely moving them, but you're still sending a signal to your fingers that you want them to move.

Only focus on your fingers and perform the movements. Remember, you're trying to only send the signal that you want the fingers to move and it's not actually important if they move or not.

Now just move your fingers and only focus on the feeling of that movement. Let yourself fall asleep. Then after about 30 seconds do a reality check.

I find it really useful to use Gingko Biloba with this technique. This is because the technique relies on focus and awareness in the moment.

You have to focus on the movement of your fingers, and that requires you to stay awake and aware during the process of falling asleep.

I've found that Gingko really helps stay aware with this technique, and actually you can use it with other things like the WILD really effectively too. It helps you maintain awareness while your body falls asleep, and you don't really need that much of it either!

Hypnagogic Imagery Technique and Claridream

This is an interesting visual technique which ca be made more effective by using dream VIVIDNESS enhancers like Claridream.

When going to sleep, relax completely, and try to remove all of your thoughts. Close your eyes. Visual images will likely appear. Do not try and focus your attention on them. Allow them to float past you as you observe them.

As you fall deeper into slumber, the images will become more complex and more similar to a dream scene. These images will eventually become vivid dream scenes.

Allow yourself to passively be drawn into the dream while keeping a sense of awareness. Do not try to involve yourself in the process of being drawn into the dream.

Conversely, too little involvement may cause you to fall asleep. If successful, you should find yourself in a lucid dream.

This might actually take a big of time to practice, because it involves a lot of mental focus and visualisation. If you struggle to see things in your minds eye, or have trouble focusing you might find this very challenging.

I'd suggest learning how to meditate before trying this. Meditation lets you improve your focus and ability to think about one particular thing for a long time. This is something that most people are naturally not very good at doing.

The one thing I found really helped with this technique though, is Claridream PRO. It lets you increase the vividness of your dreams and make everything more visual. It really helped me stay focused on the colours, and it certainly made the colours and patterns more vivid and detailed.

It's much easier to focus on something when you can actually see it, and Claridream PRO helped me see the patterns more clearly.

Dream Initiated Lucid Dream (DILD) and Alpha GPC

A Dream Induced Lucid Dream (DILD) is any dream in which you become spontaneously lucid. Your lucidity is prompted by the unreal nature of the dream. You'll consciously recognize that something isn't realistic. This realization creates lucidity.

There are many types of Dream Induced Lucid Dreams, so there are many ways to create the crucial moment of self-awareness within a dream.

Prolific lucid dreamers often have spontaneous DILDs without deliberately trying to have them. It becomes natural to understand when you are dreaming.

Certain things will trigger your inner awareness and you will realize you are dreaming. However, beginners need to spend time cultivating this mindset and habitually looking for dream signs and other reality checks.

Over time, your dreams will present the opportunities for you naturally and it is your task to move through it successfully.

This technique in itself is actually fairly easy, but I'd like to share my experiences with Alpha GPC. Alpha GPC has actually not been PROVEN to have any effect on dreams, making it an interesting one to talk about.

I've found that it can have some effect, although it's pretty difficult to know whether it's had an effect or not. The placebo effect is a powerful thing and it's even harder to study this thing yourself.

I've tried doing experiments where I'll mix up several supplements, half containing Alpha GPC and half just being empty gel capsules. I found that during that experiment, I had lucid dreams more on ALL nights!

This is because the placebo effect made me think 'this one COULD be the Alpha GPC, I wonder what my dreams will be like!'. The brain then takes over and you make yourself GET the intended result.

But there are other people who think and claim it works really well. It's one worth checking out, and seeing for yourself.

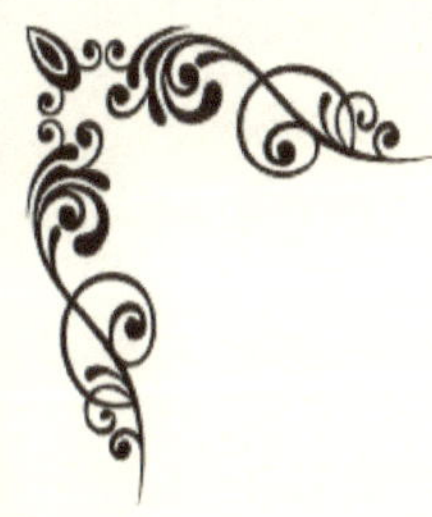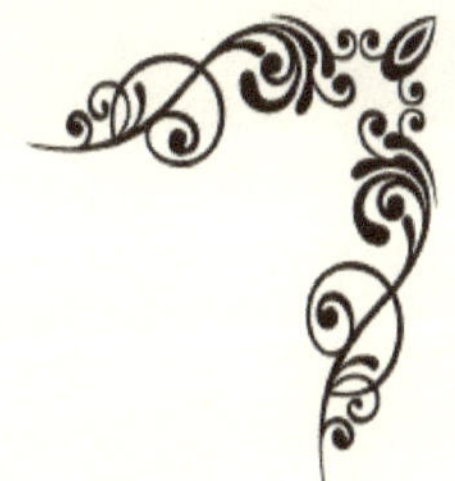

Bonus TIPS *and* TRICKS

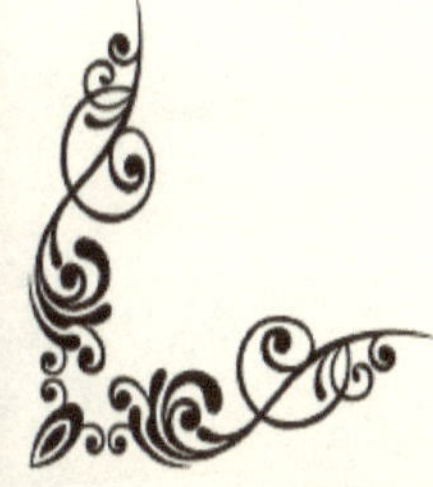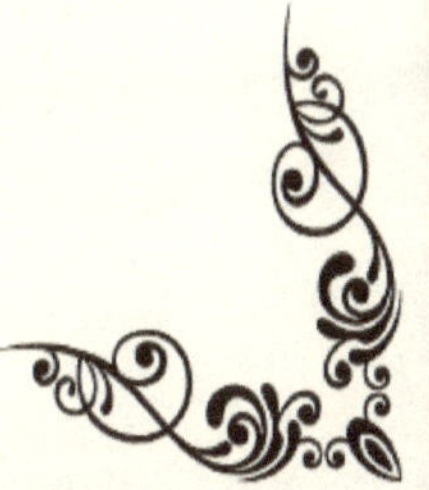

Bonus tips and tricks

This is a little bonus section which is going to have some lovely little tips and tricks for you. Firstly, remember this: Consistency is key!

Like anything you are attempting to master, it's important to be consistent in your lucid dreaming work. It's important to remember that everyone achieves results at a different rate.

Very few people are able to dream lucidly immediately and if often takes weeks or months for success. Be patient! Discipline and consistency will pay off eventually.

Journaling plays an important role for success in lucid dreams. One of the problems many people experience is a tendency to return to a full dream state after first becoming lucid. If this happens, you likely won't remember all the details of your lucid dreams.

Writing in a journal when you first wake up increases your ability to recall dreams. You will discover that many details you couldn't remember will come back to you as you write!

Journaling should be done even if you weren't able to become lucid. Dreams have a tendency to follow patterns and even dreams that seem new likely have a pattern linked to previous dreams.

The best way to recognize the pattern is to consistently journal about it and then compare dream entries over time. Once a dream pattern emerges, becoming lucid will be that much closer.

Try to write down at least one dream a day. Also consider setting an alarm every

90 minutes to wake you during REM sleep and record your dreams.

Dream journal tips and mind hacks

As you probably know, keeping a dream journal is one of the most important things you can do to lucid dream, but most people get it wrong.

There are all sorts of things you could do or write, so let's quickly go over how to best use your dream diary to have more lucid dreams.

Don't move from the position you wake up from until you have been able to remember as much detail about your dreams as you can.

The reason it is critical to remain still is because consciousness is tied into skeletal muscle activation and if refrain from moving you will retain a dream-like cognition after waking up. You may even notice that sometimes your hearing does not turn on until after you move.

Then get your dream journal and write down what you can recall.

Word the dream in the present tense

For example, "I am in my home trying to locate my wallet." Writing in present tense will keep your memory more connected to the dream events while increasing recall. Include anything you can remember including feelings and conversation. If you aren't sure about something, be clear about that fact.

It will be a temptation to skip journaling. You may be anxious to begin the rest of your day or you may think that the dream was to bother writing about. Every entry is worthwhile and you will see this over the course of time. What might seem mundane initially you will likely prove to be enlightening later.

Always record the date and TIME you woke up

Once you get into the habit of writing your dreams down, it will get easier. You may find yourself spontaneously waking after every dream and you should keep a record of what time each dream occurred.

Also think about and write down whatever events from your life which may have influenced the dream. Not only is this whole process valuable for having lucid dreams, it is also an interesting way to document your life.

Practice meditation on a regular basis

Becoming more consciously aware through this practice is one of the best ways to increase the likelihood of becoming lucid. Becoming calm and centered can only help the process—in addition to improving overall quality of life!

Listen to binaural beats during deeper meditation

Binaural beats are a type of sound that bring on altered brain states. They are very easy to use and can be found for free on the internet. In addition to making you become lucid, they also bring better sleep. You can also use them for improving energy, creativity, confidence— and a whole lot more!

Eat the right food

Food can actually be fairly important when learning to lucid dream. The food you put into your body directly affects things like mood and mental state.

Focus on improving your diet

This will improve your dreams and give you more lucidity. Also, remember to drink enough water as this has been shown to improve overall health and make thoughts more clear. Don't smoke marijuana or drink excessive alcohol because they are REM inhibitors.

Recording your dreams in audio

This is an advisable way to record your dreams. You may be too tired to turn on a light and write something in a notebook, so what can you do?

Use a voice activated recorder and speak your dreams into it for later reference.This way you don't need to use light and you can just translate the dream when you actually wake up for the day and write it down.

Also, it's not advisable to have lots of light in your room as you're falling asleep. However, natural light entering your room in the morning is very helpful. You may want to purchase blackout curtains that will stop all light entering your room but will allow some light in the morning.

Try to turn off all artificial light sources before going to sleep. This will provide a better night's sleep and make way for more dreams.

Pamper yourself before bed. When you've finished a long, treat yourself. Have a warm bath or get your partner to give you a massage. Do things that relax you.

It helps the body wind down before bed and you're more likely to fall asleep promptly. Relaxing yourself and making sure you're actually ready for bed sounds obvious, but it's often overlooked.

Make sure you spend a little bit of extra money to get a comfortable pillow. You'll really notice the difference when you buy a high quality pillow. Try not to be cheap when it comes to buying a mattress or a pillow because the quality of your sleep affects every aspect of life.

Use lots of energy during the day. Have lots of sex, exercise, work hard, etc. Make sure that by the time it comes to bedtime, you're tired out.

You want to be so tired that you can't wait to fall asleep. You will dream more easily this way and you'll feel better when you wake up because you'll have slept deeply.

Make sure your room is cool. In order for your body to go into deep sleep, body temperature is lowered significantly. In order to do this, fresh air needs to be circulating. Have you ever been camping and noticed that you wake up earlier and don't feel tired. This is because the light can easily go through the tent and activate the hormones that wake you up. It's natural and our bodies are designed to work in tandem with nature.

Try and make sure there's not much blocking air circulation under your bed. This will make it easier for your body to lower your temperature and fall asleep faster.

Having things and lots of clutter under the mattress is a common thing that people do but it STOPS them being able to sleep as well as they could.

Make sure you eat enough. Not only does this give your body the energy it needs, but it makes sure that you will operate at maximum strength. You want your body to have lots of energy and to be working properly.

By telling your friends about your commitment to lucid dreaming, you're making it more real in your psyche. Every time you tell someone about it you're giving it more power because you're talking about it.

Suddenly it becomes less abstract and more like something that's a genuine part of your life. They say the best way to learn something is to teach people what you are in the process of learning. It deepens your understanding by sharing information with others.

Have the right mindset for lucid dreams

Your mindset is very important. Let go of your fear. Lucidity is a powerful and positive tool for personal growth. What you believe and what you think will directly affect your lucid dreaming ability. Your daily thoughts will profoundly affect your success rate. Consider spending a few minutes each day affirming that you can dream lucidly and you will be successful.

Lucid dreaming is a journey; enjoy it!

Accomplishing lucidity is definitely NOT overnight thing. Nobody suddenly becomes a master of controlling dreams.

It can often take years to master the process and there will always be something new to learn. It's exciting to keep learning and discovering where the journey will take you.

Don't be in a rush! You've got your whole life to gain mastery and enjoy it.

A major reason people fail at lucid dreaming is they just try only one thing for a few days and then they promptly give up. It's usually necessary to vary techniques and to keep trying new things. Keep pushing the limits and trying new things.

If you don't keep it fresh, you will likely get stuck and feel in a rut before long. Be proactive and prevent this from happening.

Also, really want it more. Ask yourself how much you actually want to lucid dream. Many people say they want to lucid dream, but they are not fully committed to the process. They've maybe read an article or two and they want to just try it out to see what it's like.

There's a good chance they'll still have lucid dreams this way ,but to truly get results you've got to want it and work for it. Basically, you've got to be obsessed with the idea of controlling your dreams. This way you are telling your brain that you're not going to take no for an answer.

The best lucid dreaming tip ever is to believe in yourself. We all have the ability to learn lucid dreaming.

It's very real and it can be very easy to learn. You just need to know what to practice and how to practice it. Whatever you decide to do, just don't give up. Hopefully these lucid dreaming tips have helped you and inspired you in some way. May you be successful in your endeavors!

Special bonuses for book readers

As a special thank you for buying my book I'd like to share with you a secret page on my website where you can get special deals, information, and a few extra bonuses as well.

The page is updated every now and then so be sure to check it out!

This is also where you can BUY most of these supplements, at a huge discount, so check it out:

https://HowToLucid.com/BookBonus

Type it into your internet browser to see the secret page! Don't share it with anyone, it's your secret little page to help you learn more about lucid dreaming! Good luck on your journey.

Disclaimer and copyright

By reading this book you acknowledge that you're not permitted to copy, share or otherwise distribute this book and the contents of it. This is all the copyright of **_HowtoLucid.com_** (2019) and you're not permitted to share it.

The suggestions presented in this book are intended for entertainment purposes only, and you're entirely repressible for what happens when you do or do not try and or none of these suggestions.

You do not have permission to copy, edit, share or otherwise distribute this book. All the contents of this book are the copyright of **howtolucid.com** and must not be edited shared or changed. **IMPORTANT:** This book is Not intended as medical or nutritional advice, and you should consult your GP and physician before making any *changes, or taking any supplements. We are not responsible for any supplements or substances you do or do not take, and by reading this you accept full responsibility for any supplements you do or do not take.*

You should always do your own research and look at a variety of sources and research BEFORE ordering or taking any supplements and substances.